Amina Mnejja
Olfa Zoukar
Dhekra Toumi

The impact of COVID-19 on the sex life of pregnant women

Amina Mnejja
Olfa Zoukar
Dhekra Toumi

The impact of COVID-19 on the sex life of pregnant women

ScienciaScripts

Imprint

Any brand names and product names mentioned in this book are subject to trademark, brand or patent protection and are trademarks or registered trademarks of their respective holders. The use of brand names, product names, common names, trade names, product descriptions etc. even without a particular marking in this work is in no way to be construed to mean that such names may be regarded as unrestricted in respect of trademark and brand protection legislation and could thus be used by anyone.

Cover image: www.ingimage.com

This book is a translation from the original published under ISBN 978-620-6-70881-0.

Publisher:
Sciencia Scripts
is a trademark of
Dodo Books Indian Ocean Ltd. and OmniScriptum S.R.L publishing group

120 High Road, East Finchley, London, N2 9ED, United Kingdom
Str. Armeneasca 28/1, office 1, Chisinau MD-2012, Republic of Moldova, Europe
Printed at: see last page
ISBN: 978-620-8-13805-9

The impact of COVID-19 on the sex life of pregnant women

Authors :

Amina Mnejja

OlfaZoukar

DhekraToumi

Table of Contents

Introduction

Research into women's sexuality, including that of pregnant women, has recently gained in popularity.

Mental health is a state of well-being that enables people to recognise their abilities and to cope with the problems and stresses of everyday life [1].

In December 2019, an unknown cause of pneumonia was identified in Wuhan (Hubei, China), and was named acute respiratory syndrome coronavirus 2 (the cause of COVID-19) [2].

COVID-19, as the sixth public health emergency of international concern, has spread rapidly around the world since its origin [3].

The COVID-19 virus has been associated with a rapid increase in cases and deaths worldwide[4].

There is little information on the impact of this virus in

general and during pregnancy. However, there is information on illnesses associated with other pathogenic coronaviruses (e.g. Severe Acute Respiratory Syndrome (SARS) and Middle East Respiratory Syndrome (MERS)), which could be useful in understanding the impact of coronavirus during pregnancy and on mental health and well-being in general.

Previous studies have shown the widespread and profound impact of epidemics on people's mental health, which can cause new psychiatric symptoms or aggravate a previous mental illness [5].

As a public health crisis, COVID-19 has caused concern and had psychological effects on people [6].

COVID-19 is associated with a variety of problems and symptoms, from mild and asymptomatic, such as common colds, to severe symptoms such as serious respiratory illness [7].

The COVID-19 pandemic led to a number of problems and stress factors, such as restricted activities, fear of illness, loss of loved ones, life-threatening situations, unemployment, reduced income and family separation [8].

The psychosocial and economic implications of the current pandemic and its impact on community life and individual health are likely to have adverse collateral effects on general health and expose vulnerable populations to an increased risk of psychological problems [9].

Good mental health during pregnancy plays a crucial role in the progress of the pregnancy and the development of the fetus [10].

Most people do not deal with the problem of sexuality because of their gene or do not consider it to be a medical problem [11].

Materials and methods

A categorised and exhaustive bibliographic search was carried out in the literature published in PubMed, Embase, Web of Science, Scopus and the Cochrane Library in accordance with PRISMA (PreferredReporting Items for SystematicReviews and Meta-Analyses) guidelines.

The keywords entered in the various databases were :

Sexual function, Stress, Anxiety, Depression, COVID- 19, sexual relations; sexuality; pregnancy; couples, Pregnant women, Breastfeeding women, Quality of life.

After removing duplicates from a total of 163 items, 69 items were identified. Subsequently, a total of 94 items were excluded.

These were publications on murine models and other publications that were ineligible due to the availability of abstracts only or in the case of publications in languages other than English or French.

A total of 69 articles were selected for this literature review.

Results and discussion

During pregnancy, there is a progressive decline in sexual activity, interest and satisfaction. This is linked to changes in sex life, body image, neurological and hormonal systems, as well as psychological and emotional disturbances [12,13].

Throughout pregnancy, significant and profound physical and emotional changes occur in pregnant women and their partners.

Most couples remain sexually active during pregnancy.

However, some pregnant women are unsure about the safety of sexual activity and its effects on the well-being of the fetus, the health of the child and the maintenance of the pregnancy [14].

In 1966, Masters and Johnson stated that, during the first trimester of pregnancy, the sexual interest of pregnant women decreased markedly [15]. The main cause was the physiological symptoms that occur during the first trimester of pregnancy, such as drowsiness, breast pain, nausea, vomiting and mood disorders.

There are also concerns about the possibility of damage to the embryo or miscarriage as a result of sexual contact [16-19].

On the other hand, the first trimester brings changes that favour sexual relations.

Firstly, the couple no longer has to worry about contraception and protection against unwanted pregnancies [20].

During the second trimester of pregnancy, there is a visible increase in the number of sexual encounters for the vast majority of women; in addition, there is an enrichment of sexual experience, as well as an increase in sexual activity and an increase in erotic fantasies and dreams, regardless of the number of previous pregnancies [21].

This phenomenon is partly due to physical changes, such as increased congestion of the genitals and more intense lubrication of the vaginal walls as a result of hormones; however, it is also partly a psychological acclimatisation to pregnancy and acceptance of one's own appearance.

During the third trimester of pregnancy, there is a marked decrease in sexual activity, a reduction in the frequency of sexual intercourse and an alteration in the ability to experience orgasm, in both nulliparous and multiparous women, according to Eisenberg et al [22], a consequence of fear for the child or fear of premature labour.

Even today, the influence of pregnancy on female sexuality and the influence of sexual relations on the course of pregnancy are the subject of debate [2329].

Pregnancy is a critical time for women, during which prenatal psychological distress can occur [30].

In addition, anxiety and stress levels during pregnancy are linked to pregnancy complications [31].

The deleterious impact of COVID-19 on mental health has already been documented in the health sciences literature [32, 33].

On the other hand, adequate sexual functioning and intimacy are protective factors and often enhance mental health[34-36].

Sexual function is a process that involves different and diverse organs of the body and includes a woman's ability to achieve sexual arousal, orgasm and a sense of satisfaction and improves the quality of married life [37].

Despite the powerful effect of COVID-19 on overall quality of life, little information and attention is devoted to maintaining sexual health, and there is a lack of information on sexual health during COVID-19 to date [38].

Some studies have shown a relationship between sexual function and mental health [35].

Women who have an active and satisfying sexual function have greater emotional satisfaction and better mental health [39].

A review article showed that vaginal sex improves people's mental health by improving satisfaction, quality of life and well-being.

An essential component of healthcare for pregnant women during pregnancy is the assessment of sexual function [19] and mental health [40].

However, despite the importance and high prevalence of sexual dysfunction [41].

Previous studies on the Severe Acute Respiratory Syndrome (SARS) epidemic have shown that pregnant women are more likely to be anxious than non-pregnant women; these include anxiety related to infection, transmission of infection to the fetus, infection acquired during childbirth and the teratogenicity of micro-organisms and drugs.

They were afraid to go to hospitals and health centres and postponed their antenatal care [42].

Similarly, Yanting Wu et al have argued that reduced physical activity is a modifiable cause of depression during the epidemic [43].

It is very likely that infection-related pregnancy complications increase the risk of perinatal anxiety and depression [44]; moreover, they may affect the quality of life (QoL) and sexual function of the pregnant woman [45, 46].

The female sexual response cycle can be divided into four phases: baseline, arousal, orgasm and resolution.

During these phases, women may experience various sexual dysfunctions, such as a lack of drive and arousal, and an inability to reach orgasm during sexual activity.

It has also been shown that a significant reduction in sexual activity occurs with pregnancy.

Physical discomfort, fear of harming the fetus, loss of libido, physical gene, painful sexual activity, and lack of sexual attraction were among the disruptors of sexual activity during pregnancy during the COVID-19 pandemic[47].

Many symptoms of mental distress, such as depression, stress, irritability and insomnia, were reported to be higher in people who had been quarantined.

Stressors associated with quarantine include prolonged duration of quarantine, fear of infection, loss of normal life routine, reduced social activity and physical contact with others, inadequate basic supplies, lack of sufficient information, clear instructions on what to do and severe socio-economic problems [48].

Experience of previous epidemics (SARS) has shown that pregnant women suffer from high levels of anxiety, particularly those who are more emotionally vulnerable[49].

Stress and anxiety suppress the immune system [50].

Various studies have reported an association between mental morbidity during pregnancy and adverse pregnancy outcomes, such as low birth weight and preterm labour.

A possible explanation for these results is the cumulative effect of the mental burden imposed on society by COVID-19, as well as pregnancy and breastfeeding, which are mentally sensitive periods.

Given the devastating effects of anxiety and depression on the immune system, pregnancy and breastfeeding, these results underline the importance of mental health care for pregnant and breastfeeding women during the outbreak period.

The status of sexual function as a physical, emotional and mental state is an essential part of every human being and personality and the cornerstone of the couple relationship; it also has a significant impact on quality of life [51].

The vast majority of studies have shown that sexual function declines significantly during pregnancy, and this decline may continue for 3 to 6 months after delivery [52].

The present study by Yuksel et ala also demonstrated the existence of a significant decrease in sexual function in pregnant and breastfeeding women[53]. They compared frequency of sexual intercourse, desire for pregnancy and FSFI scores in women during the COVID-19 pandemic with 6 to 12 months before the pandemic. They reported higher sexual desire and frequency of intercourse, while quality of sex life was lower during the COVID-19 pandemic.

The study also revealed a significant reduction in the

number of women intending to become pregnant, which could raise concerns about its possible effects on the Icvtus [54].

Although little data is available, mid-life unemployment, anxiety about job security, worries about personal and family health, and the ability to access medical care can affect sexual desire.

Although some people may resort to sex for comfort or temporary distraction [55].

Anxiety and depression symptoms caused by "hypochondriacal preoccupation" (worry about being infected) [56] and the proven effect of anxiety and depression on sexual function [57] may explain the increase in sexual dysfunction in the COVID-19 epidemic. The results of this study by Yuksel et al showed no significant difference in sexual dysfunction between pregnant and breastfeeding women.

Both pregnancy and breastfeeding can affect sexual function through physical changes (including fatigue, back pain, dyspareunia, urinary tract infections and vaginitis), hormonal changes (altered levels of restrogenes, progesterone and prolactin levels) and psychogenic factors (such as anxiety related to childbirth and motherhood, the relationship between childbirth and motherhood, the couple's relationship, low self-esteem, sexual guilt, and specific concerns about body image and general health) [58].

Low levels of restrogen and progesterone and high levels of prolactin during breastfeeding [59] and increased blood vessels in the vagina and reduced sexual arousal during pregnancy can lead to dryness [60] .

Given the considerable impact of pregnancy [61] and breastfeeding [62] on sexual activity due to the many significant physical and mental changes, pregnant and breastfeeding women are more likely to be affected by the mental impact of COVID-19 on sexuality.

Quality of life is defined as people's perception of their position in life within their cultural and value contexts, their goals, expectations, norms and concerns [63].

With regard to factors associated with quality of life, an increased rate of depression, anxiety, sleep disorders and experience of life-threatening events have been associated with poor quality of life during pregnancy [64].

The results of the study by Yuksel et al were consistent with the results reported in the study by Lau et al, who studied the mental health and quality of life of Hong Kong residents during the SARS epidemic [65].

Han Xiao reported the effect of COVID-19 quarantine anxiety and stress on sleep quality, such as difficulty falling asleep or waking up easily [66].

Shao-YuTsai has demonstrated a high prevalence of sleep

disorders in pregnant women [67].

The results of this study by Yuksel et al indicated a lower physical QoL score throughout pregnancy compared with breastfeeding women and nonpregnant/nonbreastfeeding women, in particular with regard to reduced physical activity and physical symptoms such as nausea and vomiting, epigastralgia, reflux, breathlessness, dizziness, back pain and sleep disturbance [68].

As far as we know, there is a fairly good understanding of the correlation between pregnancy, the post-partum period and depression, but there is virtually nothing on the relationship between COVID-19 and mental health, sexual function and quality of life.

Given that the COVID-19 pandemic is still underway, these results need to be confirmed and studied in future studies on a larger population.

It should be noted that anxiety, stress and depression affect the sexual function of pregnant women; any reduction in the quality of the sexual relationship during pregnancy leads to depression [69], which indicates the reciprocal relationship between these two variables.

Sexuality is not limited to intercourse (penetration, coitus) but also simple gestures such as caressing.

Haptonomy, the science of affectivity, aims to establish a tactile relationship before birth and give the baby a sense of security that will help him or her to develop and become autonomous once born. The baby gradually responds to stimulation and an emotional relationship is gradually established between mother, father and baby in utero.

Haptonomy is more a form of support than a genuine preparation for childbirth. Based on the establishment of an emotional relationship, through caresses and gentle pressure on the abdomen, both mum and dad can encourage the child to move, to position itself in a particular way so that it is more comfortable for both of them.

Haptonomy generally begins in the fourth month of pregnancy, when the mother-to-be can feel her baby's movements. During childbirth, the father-to-be will have learned to soothe and relax you by applying gentle pressure to certain areas of the body. Some haptonomists believe that, during childbirth, the mother is also able to guide her baby thanks to the contact established during pregnancy. After the birth, parents and baby can return for a three-way session to find the right gestures to reassure the newborn.

Conclusion

In conclusion, it can be said that pregnant women and mothers in the post-partum period, as groups at high risk of mental disorders and sexual dysfunction, are more sensitive to the possible psychological effects of the coronavirus pandemic.

Therefore, it seems that more attention should be paid to mental health care services as a boon for pregnant women to combat the psychological effects of coronavirus to reduce the consequences of depression, anxiety and stress for the fretus/newborn.

Sexual satisfaction and frequency of intercourse decrease in couples during pregnancy. Pregnancy does not change partnerships, but sexual problems during pregnancy can have a negative impact on the relationship and constitute additional stress factors for couples.

Medical staff should be trained to assess sexual difficulties in people during pregnancy, in order to provide reliable education and raise couples' awareness of sexual and reproductive health.

In conclusion, a woman who is prepared for childbirth, or rather a couple who are well cared for during pregnancy, can maintain a normal sex life without any decline during pregnancy and in the post-partum period.

References

1. Friedli L. Mental health, resilience and inequalities, vol. 31. Copenhagen: World Health Organization. Retrieved March; 2009. p. 2018.

2. WHO. WHO Statement regarding cluster of pneumonia cases in Wuhan, China: WHO; 9 January 2020 [Available from: https://www.who.int/china/news/detai l/09-01 -2020-who-state ment-regar ding-clust er-of-pneumonia-cases -inwuhan -china .

3. Organization WH. WHO Director-General'sremarks at the media briefingon 2019-nCoV on 11 February 2020. Internet] World Health Organization.2020.

4. Muniyappa R, Gubbi S. COVID-19 pandemic, coronaviruses, and diabetes mellitus. Am J Physiol Endocrinol Metab. 2020;318(5): E736-E41. https://doi.org/10.1152/ajpendo.00124.2020.

5. Hall RC, Hall RC, Chapman MJ. The 1995 Kikwit

Ebola outbreak: lessons hospitals and physicians can apply to future viral epidemics. Gen Hosp Psychiatry. 2008;30(5):446-52.

6. Bao Y, Sun Y, Meng S, Shi J, Lu L. 2019-nCoV epidemic: address mental health care to empower society. Lancet.2020;395(10224):e37-8.

7. Rasmussen SA, Smulian JC, Lednicky JA, Wen TS, Jamieson DJ. Coronavirus disease 2019 (COVID-19) and pregnancy: what obstetricians need to know. Am J Obstet Gynecol. 2020;222(5): 415-26.

8. Bedford J, Enria D, Giesecke J, Heymann DL, Ihekweazu C, Kobinger G, et al. COVID-19: towards scontrolling of a pandemic. Lancet. 2020;395(10229): 1015-8. https://doi.org/10.1016/S0140-673 6(20)3 0673 - 5.

9. Lee DT, Sahota D, Leung TN, Yip AS, Lee FF, Chung TK. Psychological responses of pregnant women to an

infectious outbreak: a case-control study of the 2003 SARS outbreak in Hong Kong. J Psychosom Res. 2006; 61(5):707-13. https://doi.org/10.1016Zj.jpsychores.2006.08.005.

10. Guszkowska M, Langwald M, Zaremba A, Dudziak D. The correlates of mental health of well-educated polish women in the first pregnancy. J Ment Health. 2014;23(6):328-32. https ://doi.or g/10.3109/09638237.2 014.971144.

11. Zemishlany Z, Weizman A. The impact of mental illness on sexual dysfunction. Sexual dysfunction. 29: Karger Publishers; 2008. p. 89-106.

12. Rossi, M.A.; Impett, E.A.; Dawson, S.J.; Vannier, S.; Kim, J.; Rosen, N.O. A Longitudinal Investigation of Couples' Sexual Growth and Destiny Beliefs in the Transition to Parenthood. Arch. Sex. Behav. 2022, 117. [CrossRef] [PubMed]

13. Sassine, D.; Ghulmiyyah, L.; Atallah, S.; Ghieh, D.; Saleh, N.; Slim, S.; Rameh, G. Sexual Changes during Pregnancy in a Middle-Eastern Population. Sex. Cult. 2020, 24, 1232-1251. [CrossRef]

14. Aydin, M.; Cayonu, N.; Kadihasanoglu, M.; Irkilata, L. ; Atilla, M.K.; Kendirci, M. Comparison of sexual functions in pregnant and non-pregnant women. Urol. J. 2015, 12, 2339-2344.

15. Jawed-Wessel, S.; Sevick, E. The Impact of Pregnancy and Childbirth on Sexual Behaviors: A Systematic Review. J. Sex Res. 2017, 54, 411-423. [CrossRef]

16. Eepecka-Klusek, C.; Syty, K.; Pilewska-Kozak, A.B.; Jakiel, G. Sense of own attractiveness among women in advanced pregnancy. Prog. Health Sci. 2015, 5, 7-13.

17. Lew-Starowicz, Z.; Skrzypulec, V. (Eds.) Podstawy Seksuologii; PZWL: Warszawa, Poland, 2010.

18. Fuchs, A.; Czech, I.; Sikora, J.; Fuchs, P.; Lorek, M .; Skrzypulec-Plinta, V.; Drosdzol-Cop, A. Sexual Functioning in Pregnant Women. Int. J. Environ. Res. Public Health 2019, 16, 4216. [CrossRef]

19. Jawed-Wessel, S.; Santo, J.; Irwin, J. Sexual Activity and Attitudes as Predictors of Sexual Satisfaction during Pregnancy: A Multi-Level Model Describing the Sexuality of Couples in the First 12 Weeks. Arch. Sex. Behav. 2019, 48, 843-854. [CrossRef]

20. Bartellas, E.; Crane, J.M.G.; Daley, M.; Bennett, K.A.; Hutchens, D. Sexuality and sexual activity in pregnancy. BJOG Int. J. Obstet. Gynaecol. 2000, 107, 964-968. [CrossRef] [PubMed]

21. An" gin, A.D.; Ozkaya, E.; £etin, M.; Gün, I.; Sakin, O.; Ertekin, L.T.; Denizli, R.; Koyuncu, K.; Akalin, E.E. Comparison of female

22. Eisenberg, A.; Murkoff, H.; Hathaway, S.WO

czekiwaniu na Dziecko: Poradnikdla Przyszlych Matek i *Ojcbw*; Rebis, DomWydawniczy: Pozna'n, Poland, 2002.

23. Obrochta, C.A.; Chambers, C.; Bandoli, G. Psychological distress in pregnancy and postpartum. Women Birth 2020, 33, 583-591. [CrossRef] [PubMed]

24. Fitzpatrick, E.T.; Kolbuszewska, M.T.; Dawson, S.J. Perinatal Sexual Dysfunction: The Importance of the Interpersonal Context. Curr. Sex. HealthRep. 2021, 13, 55-65. [CrossRef]

25. Lorenz, T.K.; Ramsdell, E.L.; Brock, R.L. Communication changes the effects of sexual pain on sexual frequency in the pregnancy to postpartum transition. J. Psychosom. Obstet. Gynecol. 2020, 2020, 1-8. [CrossRef]

26. Carpenter, E.; Everett, B.G.; Greene, M.Z.; Haider, S.; Hendrick, C.E.; Higgins, J.A. Pregnancy (im) possibilities: Identifying factors that influence sexual minority women's

pregnancy desires. Soc. Work Health Care 2020, 59, 180-198. [CrossRef]

27. Masters, W.H.; Johnson, V.E. Human Sexual Response Little; Brown: Boston, MA, USA, 1966.

28. Kyndely, K. The Sexuality of Women in Pregnancy and Postpartum: A Review. Med. Asp. Hum. Sex 1978, 7, 28-32. [CrossRef]

29. Imieli'nski, K.; Imieli'nski, C. Sexual problems among women during pregnancy. In Sexologists from Criminal Law to the Gynecology; Imieli'nski, K., Ed.; Polska Akademia Wiedzy Seksuologicznej: Warszawa, Poland, 1997; pp. 211-214.

30. Effati-Daryani F, Mohammad-Alizadeh-Charandabi S, Zarei S, et al. Depression, anxiety and stress in the various trimesters of pregnancy in women referring to Tabriz health centres, 2016. Int J Cult Ment Health. 2018;11(4):513-21.

https://doi.org/10.1080/17542863.2018.1438484.

31. Kingston D, Tough S, Whit field H. Prenatal and postpartum maternal psychological distress and infant development: asystematic review. Child Psychiatry Hum Dev. 2012;43(5):683-714. https://doi.org/10.1007/s10578- 012-0291-4.

32. Wang C, Pan R, Wan X, Tan Y, Xu L, Ho CS, et al. Immediate psychological responses and associated factors during the initial stage of the 2019 coronavirus disease (COVID-19) epidemic among the general population in China. Int J Environ Res Public Health. 2020; 17(5): 1729.

33. Xiao H, Zhang Y, Kong D, Li S, Yang N. The effects of social support on sleep quality of medical staff treating patients with coronavirus disease 2019 (COVID-19) in January and February 2020 in China. Med SciMonit. 2020;26:e923549-1.

34. Galbally M, Watson SJ, Permezel M, Lewis AJ.

Depression across pregnancy and the postpartum, antidepressant use and the association with female sexual function. Psychol Med. 2019;49(9): 1490-9.https://doi.org/10.1017/ S0033291718002040.

35. Nik-Azin A, Nainian MR, Zamani M, Bavojdan MR, Motlagh MJ. Evaluation of sexual function, quality of life, and mental and physical health in pregnant women. J Family Reprod Health. 2013;7(4):171-6.

36. Lteif Y, Kesrouani A, Richa S. Depressive syndromes during pregnancy: prevalence and risk factors. J Gynecol Obstet Biol Reprod (Paris). 2005;34(3 Pt 1):262-9. https://doi.org/10.1016/S0368- 2315(05)82745-0.

37. Leite APL, Campos AAS, Dias ARC, Amed AM, De Souza E, Camano L. Prevalence of sexual dysfunction during pregnancy. Rev Assoc Méd Bras. 2009;55(5):563-8. https://doi.org/10.1590/S0104-42302009000500020.

38. Ibarra FP, Mehrad M, Mauro MD, Godoy MFP, Cruz

EG, Nilforoushzadeh MA, et al. Impact of the COVID-19 pandemic on the sexual behavior of the population. The vision of the east and the west. Int Braz J Urol. 2020; 46 (suppl 1): 104-12. https://doi.org/10.1590/s1677-5538.ibju.2020.s116.

39. Rosen RC, Bachmann GA. Sexual well-being, happiness, and satisfaction, in women: the case for a new conceptual paradigm. J Sex Marital Ther. 2008; 34(4):291-7. https://doi.org/10.1080/00926230802096234.

40. Van Bussel JC, Spitz B, Demyttenaere K. Women's mental health before, during, and after pregnancy: a population-based controlled cohort study. Birth. 2006;33(4):297-302. https://doi.org/10.1111/j.1523-536X.2006.00122.x.

41. Daud S, Zahid AZM, Mohamad M, Abdullah B, Mohamad NAN. Prevalence of sexual dysfunction in pregnancy. Arch Obstet Gynaecol. 2019;300(5): 127985.

https://doi.org/10.1007/s00404-019-05273-y.

42. Lee DT, Sahota D, Leung TN, Yip AS, Lee FF, Chung TK. Psychological responses of pregnant women to an infectious outbreak: a case-control study of the 2003 SARS outbreak in Hong Kong. J Psychosom Res.2006;61(5):707-13.

43. Wu Y, Zhang C, Liu H, Duan C, Li C, Fan J, *et al.* Perinatal depressive and anxiety symptoms of pregnant women along with COVID-19 outbreak in China. Am J ObstGynecol. 2020;223(2):240.e1-e9.

44. Dowse E, Chan S, Ebert L, Wynne O, Thomas S, Jones D, *et al*. Impact of perinatal depression and anxiety on birth out comes: are tros pective data analysis. Matern Child Health J. 2020;24(6):718-26.

45. Basson R, Gilks T. Women's sexual dysfunction associated with psychiatric disorders and their treatment. Womens Health. 2018;14:1745506518762664.

46. Mourady D, Richa S, Karam R, Papazian T, Moussa FH, El Osta N, *et al.* Associations between quality of life, physical activity, worry, depression and insomnia: a cross-sectional designed study in healthy pregnant women. PLoS ONE. 2017;12(5):e0178181.

47 Orji EO, Ogunlola IO, Fasubaa OB. Sexuality among pregnant women in South West Nigeria. J Obstet Gynaecol. 2002;22(02): 166-168. Doi: 10.1080/01443610120113319

48. Brooks SK, Webster RK, Smith LE, Woodland L, Wessely S, Greenberg N, *etal.* The psychological impact of quarantine and how to reduceit: rapidreview of the evidence. Lancet. 2020;395:912.

49. Ng J, Sham A, Leng TP, Fung S. Pregnant Women's Perceptions on Severe Acute Respiratory Syndrome (SARS) risk.

50. Seger strom SC, Miller GE. Psychological stress and the humanimmune system: a meta-analytic study of 30 years of inquiry. Psychol Bull.2004;130(4):601.

51. Basson R. Women's sexual dysfunction: revised and expanded definitions. CMAJ. 2005;172(10):1327-33.

52. Serati M, Salvatore S, Siesto G, Cattoni E, Zanirato M, Khullar V, *et al.* Female sexual function during pregnancy and after child birth. J Sex Med.2010;7(8):2782-90.

53. Yuksel B, Ozgor F. Effect of the COVID-19 pandemic on female sexual behavior. Int J Gynecol Obstettr. 2020;150(1):102-98.

54. Liu S, Han J, Xiao D, Ma C, Chen B. A report on the reproductive health of women after the massive 2008 Wenchuane arthquake. Int J Gynecol Obstettr. 2010;108(2):161-4.

55. Gunter J. The New York Times (March 30, 2020)

Coronavirus and Sex: Questions and Answers [Available from:
https ://www.nytimes.com/2020/03/30/style /sex-coron aviru s-quest ions-answe rs.html.

56. Huang Y, Zhao N. Generalized anxiety disorder, depressive symptoms and sleep quality during COVID- 19 outbreak in China: a web-based cross sectional survey. Psychiatry Res. 2020;288:112954.

57. Brotto L, Atallah S, Johnson-Agbakwu C, Rosen baum T, Abdo C, Byers ES,*et al.* Psychological and interpersonal dimensions of sexual function and dysfunction. J Sex Med. 2016;13(4):538-71.

58. Johnson CE. Sexual health during pregnancy and the postpartum (CME).J Sex Med. 2011;8(5):1267-84.

59. Reamy KJ, White SE. Sexuality in the puerperium: are view. Arch SexBehav. 1987;16(2):165-86.

60. Jamali S, Mosalanejad L. Sexualdysfnction in Iranian pregnant women. Iran J Reprod Med. 2013; 11(6):479-86.

61. Bartellas E, Crane JM, Daley M, Bennett KA, Hutchens D. Sexuality and sexual activity in pregnancy. BJOG: Int J Obstet Gynaecol. 2000;107(8):964-8.

62. Leeman LM, Rogers RG. Sex after child birth: postpartum sexual function. Obstet Gynecol. 2012; 119(3):647-55.

63. World Health Organization. Division of Mental H, Prevention of Substance A. WHOQOL: measuring quality of life. Geneva: World Health Organization; 1997

64. Kazemi F, Nahidi F, Kariman N. Assessment scales, associated factor sand the quality of life score in pregnantwomen in Iran. Glob J Health Sci.2016;8(11):127-39.

65. Lau J, Yang X, Tsui H, Kim J. Monitoring community responses to the SARS epidemic in Hong Kong: from day

10 to day 62. J Epidemiol Community Health. 2003;57(11):864-70.

66. Xiao H, Zhang Y, Kong D, Li S, Yang N. Social capital and sleep quality in individual swho self-isolated for 14 days during the coronavirus disease2019 (COVID-19) outbreak in January 2020 in China. Med Sci Monit: Int Med J Exp Clin Res. 2020;26:e923921- 31.

67. Tsai S-Y, Lee P-L, Lin J-W, Lee C-N. Cross-sectional and longitudinal Associations betweens leep and health-related quality of life in pregnant women: a prospective observational study. Int J Nurs Stud. 2016;56:45-53.

68. Lagadec N, Steinecker M, Kapassi A, Magnier AM, Chastang J, Robert S, *etal.* Factors influencing the quality of life of pregnant women: asystematic review. BMC Pregnancy Childbirth. 2018;18(1):455.

69. Mazinani R, Akbari Mehr M, Kaskian A, Kashanian M. Evaluation of prevalence of sexual dysfunctions and its

related factors in women. Razi J Med Sci. 2013;19(105):59-66.

Summary

Introduction:

Mental health is a state of well-being that enables people to recognise their abilities and to cope with the problems and stresses of everyday life [1].

Materials and methods :

This is a literature review taking 69 articles published between 1987 and 2022 from pub med, googlescolar, google.

Results and discussion :

During pregnancy, there is a progressive decline in sexual activity, interest and satisfaction. This is linked to changes in sex life, body image, neurological and hormonal systems, as well as psychological and emotional disturbances [12,13].

Women who have an active and satisfying sexual function

have greater emotional satisfaction and better mental health [39].

Sexuality is not limited to intercourse (penetration, coitus) but also simple gestures such as caressing.

Conclusion:

It can be said that pregnant women and mothers in the post-partum period, who are at high risk of mental disorders and sexual dysfunction, are more sensitive to the possible psychological effects of the pandemic.

Biography

Amina Mnejja, resident in obstetrics and gynaecology Passionate about the internet, reading and scientific research.

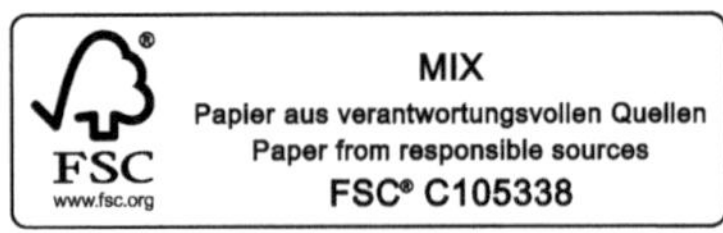

Printed by Books on Demand GmbH, Norderstedt / Germany